Exploring Contemporary Fitness Trends in America

"Unveiling the Pulse of Fitness: A Dive into Modern Exercise Trends in America"

BY

SMITH ROBERTSON

COPYRIGHT PAGE

© [2024] by Smith Robertson

TABLE OF CONTENTS:

   - Analysis of group fitness classes
   - Social and motivational aspects
   - Examples of trending group workouts

7. **Nutrition and Fitness Integration**
   - Importance of nutrition in achieving fitness goals
   - Trends in fitness-oriented diets
   - Tips for combining nutrition and exercise
effectively

8. **Recovery and Wellness Techniques**
   - Focus on recovery as an essential part of fitness
   - Overview of recovery methods
   - Importance of rest and sleep in the fitness
journey

9. **Virtual Fitness Experiences**
   - Impact of technology on virtual fitness
   - Online fitness classes and platforms
   - Pros and cons of virtual fitness experiences

10. **Conclusion**
   - Recap of key fitness trends discussed
   - Encouragement for readers to explore and find
what suits their preferences

This table of contents provides a structured
approach to exploring various fitness trends,
offering a comprehensive guide for your audience.

CHAPTER 1

INTRODUCTION:

In recent years, the fitness landscape in America has undergone a remarkable transformation, reflecting changing attitudes towards health and wellness. The traditional approach to fitness has evolved into a dynamic and diverse ecosystem, shaped by emerging trends and technologies. Staying updated on these fitness trends is not merely a matter of keeping pace with the latest fads; it's a crucial aspect of maintaining a healthy lifestyle and achieving holistic well-being.

The Evolving Fitness Landscape

Historically, fitness in America has been synonymous with gym memberships, weightlifting, and cardio routines. However, the modern fitness scene has transcended these conventional boundaries. Today, individuals are embracing a plethora of exercise modalities, from high-intensity interval training (HIIT) and functional fitness to mindfulness-based practices like yoga and meditation.

Moreover, the integration of technology has revolutionized the way we approach fitness. Wearable devices, fitness apps, and virtual training programs have become integral tools for individuals seeking personalized and data-driven workout experiences. This tech-driven shift not only enhances the effectiveness of workouts but also fosters a sense of accountability and motivation.

Significance of Staying Updated:

Understanding and incorporating the latest fitness trends is not merely a pursuit of novelty; it's a strategic investment in one's health. As scientific research advances, our understanding of the human body and optimal training methods evolves. Staying updated ensures that individuals can benefit from the most efficient and scientifically proven approaches to fitness.

Moreover, fitness trends often reflect broader societal shifts towards wellness and self-care. The emphasis on mental health, for instance, has led to an increased focus on mind-body exercises and holistic well-being practices. By staying informed, individuals can align their fitness routines with these overarching principles, fostering a more comprehensive approach to health.

Adaptability and Diversity:

The fitness landscape's constant evolution also underscores the importance of adaptability. What works for one person may not be suitable for another, and recognizing this diversity is key to creating inclusive and sustainable fitness habits. By staying informed about emerging trends, individuals can explore a variety of options, tailoring their fitness routines to align with personal preferences and goals.

Furthermore, staying updated on fitness trends facilitates social engagement. Participating in group classes or online communities centered around a particular trend not only enhances motivation but also provides a sense of belonging. This social aspect of fitness can significantly contribute to long-term adherence and overall well-being.

In conclusion, the evolving fitness landscape in America demands a proactive approach to staying informed about the latest trends. Beyond being a means of keeping up with the times, this awareness is a powerful tool for optimizing health and well-being. By embracing diversity, leveraging technology, and understanding the broader societal shifts, individuals can craft personalized and effective fitness routines that contribute to a healthier, more fulfilling life. Staying updated is not just a choice; it's a commitment to a journey of continuous improvement and vitality.

Chapter 2

HIGH-INTENSITY INTERVAL TRAINING (HIIT)

High-Intensity Interval Training (HIIT) has emerged as a popular and effective exercise regimen, captivating fitness enthusiasts with its time-efficient approach and promising results. In this chapter, we will delve into the explanation of HIIT, explore its popularity, provide sample workout routines, and discuss the myriad benefits along with important considerations.

Explanation of HIIT:

HIIT is a form of cardiovascular exercise that alternates between short bursts of intense activity and periods of rest or low-intensity exercise. The key is to push your body to near maximum effort during the high-intensity intervals, followed by a brief recovery or lower-intensity phase. This cycle is repeated throughout the workout, creating a potent cardiovascular and metabolic stimulus.

The rationale behind HIIT lies in its ability to elevate the heart rate quickly and challenge the body's energy systems. This dynamic approach not only burns calories during the workout but also induces the "afterburn" effect, scientifically known as excess post-exercise oxygen consumption (EPOC). This means that the body continues to burn calories at an elevated rate post-exercise, aiding in fat loss and improved metabolic health.

Popularity of HIIT:

HIIT's rise to popularity can be attributed to several factors. First and foremost, it addresses the time constraints that many individuals face in their busy lives. A typical HIIT session can be completed in 15-30 minutes, making it a feasible option for those with demanding schedules.
Moreover, HIIT's effectiveness in burning fat and improving cardiovascular fitness has been supported by numerous scientific studies. This evidence has resonated with people looking for efficient ways to achieve their fitness goals without spending hours in the gym. The versatility of HIIT, allowing it to be adapted to various fitness levels and preferences, has also contributed to its widespread appeal.

Sample HIIT Workout Routines:

1. **Tabata Training:**
   - 20 seconds of high-intensity exercise (e.g., sprinting, burpees)
   - 10 seconds of rest
   - Repeat for a total of 4 minutes

2. **Pyramid HIIT**:
   - 30 seconds of high-intensity exercise
   - 15 seconds of rest
   - Increase intensity for the next round, then decrease
   - Repeat for 15-20 minutes

3. **The 5-5-5 HIIT:**
   - 5 minutes of warm-up
   - 5 cycles of 1-minute high-intensity exercise followed by 1 minute of rest
   - 5 minutes of cool-down

These are just a few examples, and the beauty of HIIT lies in its adaptability. Exercises can include anything from sprinting and jumping jacks to bodyweight exercises like squats and push-ups.

Benefits and Considerations:

Benefits:

***Efficient Time Use**: HIIT workouts can be completed in a fraction of the time compared to traditional steady-state cardio.

***Fat Loss:** The intensity of HIIT contributes to increased calorie burn and fat loss.

***Cardiovascular Health**: HIIT has been shown to improve cardiovascular health, including heart health and blood pressure.

***Metabolic Boost:** The afterburn effect leads to an elevated metabolism post-exercise.

Considerations:

***Intensity**: Beginners should gradually increase intensity to avoid overexertion and injury.

***Recovery**: Sufficient rest is crucial; overtraining can lead to burnout and decreased performance.

***Individual Differences**: HIIT may not be suitable for everyone; individuals with certain health conditions should consult a healthcare professional before starting.

In conclusion, High-Intensity Interval Training is a potent and time-efficient approach to fitness, offering a myriad of benefits. Whether you're a seasoned athlete or a fitness novice, incorporating HIIT into your routine can provide a challenging and rewarding workout experience. As with any exercise program, it's essential to listen to your body, progress at a comfortable pace, and consult with a fitness professional if needed.

Chapter 3

WEARABLE FITNESS TECHNOLOGY: REVOLUTIONIZING HEALTH AND WELLNESS

In the dynamic landscape of health and wellness, wearable fitness technology has emerged as a powerful force, reshaping the way individuals engage with their physical activity and overall well-being. This article provides a comprehensive overview of fitness trackers and smartwatches, exploring their functionalities, impact on user behavior, and the evolving role they play in promoting a healthier lifestyle.

The Rise of Wearable Fitness Technology

The advent of wearable fitness technology marked a paradigm shift in how people monitor and manage their fitness goals. Fitness trackers and smartwatches, the cornerstones of this revolution, are equipped with an array of sensors and features designed to track various aspects of physical activity and health.

1. Fitness Trackers: Beyond Step Counting

Fitness trackers, such as Fitbit and Garmin, gained popularity for their ability to monitor daily steps, calories burned, and sleep patterns. However, their capabilities have expanded significantly. Modern fitness trackers now include heart rate monitors, GPS tracking, and even advanced metrics like oxygen saturation levels. This holistic approach provides users with a more comprehensive understanding of their overall health.

2. Smartwatches: The All-in-One Solution

Smartwatches, exemplified by the Apple Watch and Samsung Galaxy Watch series, go beyond fitness tracking. They integrate seamlessly into daily life, offering features like notifications, music control, and third-party apps. With built-in sensors, smartwatches deliver accurate fitness data while offering a wide range of functionalities, transforming them into indispensable companions for both health and lifestyle management.

FUNCTIONALITIES AND FEATUREs*

1. Activity Tracking and Monitoring

Both fitness trackers and smartwatches excel in monitoring various physical activities. They can distinguish between walking, running, cycling, and more, providing users with detailed insights into their workouts. Real-time data, such as heart rate and distance covered, enables immediate adjustments to optimize performance and prevent overexertion.

2. Heart Rate Monitoring

Accurate heart rate monitoring is a pivotal feature, allowing users to gauge their cardiovascular health during workouts and daily activities. Continuous monitoring also enables the detection of irregularities, potentially alerting users to underlying health issues.

3. Sleep Tracking

Understanding the importance of sleep in overall well-being, wearable fitness technology has integrated advanced sleep tracking features. Users receive detailed analyses of their sleep patterns, helping them make informed decisions to improve the quality and duration of their rest.

IMPACT ON USER BEHAVIOR

1. Motivation and Accountability

One of the key benefits of wearable fitness technology is its ability to motivate users. The gamification of fitness, with features like step challenges and achievement badges, transforms physical activity into an engaging and rewarding experience. Additionally, the constant monitoring fosters a sense of accountability, encouraging individuals to stay consistent with their health goals.

2. Personalized Insights

The data collected by fitness trackers and smartwatches allow for personalized insights. Machine learning algorithms analyze trends and patterns, providing users with tailored recommendations for workouts, nutrition, and recovery. This personalized approach enhances the effectiveness of fitness routines, making them more attuned to individual needs.

The Future of Wearable Fitness Technology

As technology continues to advance, the future of wearable fitness technology holds exciting possibilities. Integrations with artificial intelligence, improved sensor accuracy, and the development of new health metrics are on the horizon. Moreover, collaborations between wearable tech companies and healthcare providers could lead to a more integrated approach to preventive healthcare.

Lastly, Wearable fitness technology has transcended its initial role as a mere accessory, evolving into an indispensable tool for individuals striving to lead healthier lives. The amalgamation of fitness trackers and smartwatches has not only reshaped the way we approach physical activity but has also fostered a culture of proactively managing our well-being. As these devices continue to evolve, the synergy between technology and health is poised to redefine our understanding of personal fitness and pave the way for a healthier and more connected future.

NAVIGATING THE IMPACT ON PERSONAL FITNESS GOALS

In the fast-paced and demanding world we live in, personal fitness goals have become paramount in maintaining overall well-being. However, various factors can impact these goals, ranging from lifestyle changes to external pressures. Understanding and navigating these influences is crucial for individuals striving to achieve and maintain their desired level of fitness.

Lifestyle Changes:

One of the primary influences on personal fitness goals is lifestyle changes. Shifts in daily routines, such as starting a new job, becoming a parent, or relocating, can significantly impact the time and energy available for fitness pursuits. Adapting to these changes requires a flexible mindset and the ability to modify workout routines to fit the current lifestyle.

Nutritional Habits:

Another critical aspect of personal fitness is nutrition. Changes in dietary habits, whether intentional or unintentional, can either support or hinder fitness goals. Adopting a balanced diet that aligns with individual fitness objectives is essential. Consulting with a nutritionist can provide valuable insights into crafting a diet that fuels workouts and promotes overall health.

Psychological Well-being:

The mind plays a pivotal role in personal fitness journeys. Stress, anxiety, and other mental health factors can impact motivation and commitment to fitness goals. Incorporating mindfulness practices, such as meditation or yoga, can contribute to a balanced mental state, fostering a positive attitude towards exercise.

Social Influences:

The social environment can significantly affect personal fitness goals. Peer pressure, societal expectations, or the influence of friends and family can either motivate or deter individuals from staying on track with their fitness routines. Building a supportive network and communicating fitness goals can help individuals navigate external influences and garner encouragement.

Technology and Fitness:

The advent of technology has transformed the fitness landscape. While fitness apps, wearables, and online communities provide valuable resources, they can also be overwhelming. Striking a balance between leveraging technology for support and avoiding information overload is crucial for maintaining focus on personal fitness goals.

Age and Physical Limitations:

As individuals age, their bodies may undergo changes that affect their fitness capabilities. Understanding and adapting to these changes is essential for setting realistic fitness goals. Consulting with healthcare professionals or fitness experts can help tailor workout plans to accommodate age-related considerations and physical limitations.

Balancing Cardiovascular and Strength Training:

Achieving a well-rounded fitness routine involves balancing cardiovascular and strength training exercises. Some individuals may favor one over the other, impacting overall fitness outcomes. Striking a balance between cardio and strength workouts ensures comprehensive fitness development, addressing both endurance and muscle strength.

Navigating the impact on personal fitness goals requires a holistic approach that considers lifestyle changes, nutritional habits, mental well-being, social influences, technological advancements, and age-related considerations. By understanding these factors and making informed decisions, individuals can adapt their fitness routines to align with their evolving circumstances. Flexibility, resilience, and a commitment to overall well-being are key components in achieving and sustaining personal fitness goals in the face of life's dynamic challenges.

NOTABLE TRENDS IN FITNESS TECHNOLOGY

Fitness technology has undergone a remarkable transformation in recent years, revolutionizing the way individuals approach health and wellness. From wearable devices to virtual fitness platforms, the industry continues to evolve rapidly, integrating cutting-edge advancements to enhance the overall fitness experience. Here are some notable trends that have taken the fitness tech world by storm.

1. **Wearable Fitness Trackers**
Wearable fitness trackers have become ubiquitous, offering users real-time data on their physical activity, heart rate, sleep patterns, and more. These devices have evolved beyond simple step counters, incorporating advanced sensors and algorithms to provide comprehensive health insights. Integration with smartphones allows users to track their progress, set goals, and stay motivated, fostering a more proactive approach to personal fitness.

2. **Smart Clothing and Biometric Apparel**
The intersection of fashion and technology has given rise to smart clothing designed to monitor and enhance athletic performance. Biometric apparel incorporates sensors directly into clothing, measuring metrics such as muscle activity, posture, and body temperature. This innovation not only provides valuable data for users but also eliminates the need for additional devices, offering a seamless and integrated fitness experience.

3. **Virtual and Augmented Reality Fitness**
The rise of virtual and augmented reality (VR and AR) has made its way into the fitness realm, transforming traditional workout routines into immersive and engaging experiences. VR workouts transport users to virtual environments, providing a novel way to stay active and motivated. AR, on the other hand, overlays digital information onto the

real world, allowing users to interact with virtual elements while exercising in their own space.

4. AI-Powered Personalized Workouts

Artificial intelligence (AI) is playing a pivotal role in tailoring fitness routines to individual needs. Advanced algorithms analyze user data, including fitness levels, preferences, and performance history, to create personalized workout plans. This not only optimizes the effectiveness of each session but also keeps users challenged and motivated by adapting to their evolving capabilities.

5. Fitness Apps and Online Platforms

The proliferation of fitness apps and online platforms has democratized access to a wide range of workouts and wellness resources. These applications offer guided exercises, nutritional guidance, and community support, making it easier for individuals to pursue their fitness goals from the comfort of their homes. The convenience and flexibility provided by these platforms have reshaped the landscape of traditional gym memberships.

6. Recovery Tech: Massage Guns and Compression Therapy

Recovery is an integral part of any fitness regimen, and technology has introduced innovative solutions to expedite the process. Massage guns, utilizing percussive therapy, have gained popularity for their ability to alleviate muscle soreness and improve recovery. Compression therapy devices, ranging from sleeves to full-body suits, aid in reducing inflammation and enhancing blood circulation, contributing to faster recovery times.

7. Health and Wellness Wearables Beyond Fitness

The integration of health monitoring features into everyday wearables expands their utility beyond fitness tracking. Devices now offer capabilities such as continuous blood pressure monitoring, ECG measurements, and stress tracking. This shift towards holistic health monitoring aligns with a broader societal focus on overall well-being, positioning these wearables as essential tools for proactive health management.

In conclusion, the trends in fitness technology are indicative of a dynamic and constantly evolving landscape. As technology continues to advance, the fitness industry can expect further innovations that enhance the accessibility, personalization, and effectiveness of fitness experiences. Whether through AI-driven workouts, immersive virtual environments, or multifunctional wearables, these advancements contribute to a future where individuals have unprecedented control over their health and fitness journeys.

Chapter 4

MIND-BODY CONNECTION: YOGA AND MEDITATION

In recent years, there has been a noticeable surge in the interest surrounding holistic fitness, with individuals seeking a more integrated approach to well-being that goes beyond physical exercise. Central to this movement is the profound connection between the mind and body, and two practices that have gained widespread popularity for fostering this connection are yoga and meditation.

Yoga: A Union of Mind and Body

Originating in ancient India, yoga is not merely a physical practice but a philosophy that emphasizes the union of mind, body, and spirit. The physical postures (asanas) in yoga are just one aspect of a comprehensive system aimed at achieving balance and harmony.

Asanas, combined with breath control (pranayama) and meditation, create a holistic approach to fitness. The various styles of yoga, from the vigorous Vinyasa to the more meditative Yin, cater to different preferences and needs, providing a versatile toolkit for practitioners.

Yoga's impact extends beyond the physical realm. Regular practice has been linked to improved mental well-being, stress reduction, and increased self-awareness. It encourages mindfulness, allowing individuals to be present in the moment and cultivate a deeper understanding of their thoughts and emotions.

Meditation: Cultivating Mental Fitness

Meditation, another ancient practice that has found its place in modern lifestyles, is the art of training the mind to achieve a state of focused awareness. This practice comes in various forms, such as mindfulness meditation, transcendental meditation, and loving-kindness meditation.

Mindfulness meditation, in particular, has gained popularity for its simplicity and effectiveness. It involves paying attention to the present moment without judgment, often through focusing on the breath or observing thoughts. Research suggests that regular meditation can lead to structural changes in the brain associated with improved attention and emotional regulation.

Meditation serves as a complement to yoga, enhancing the mind-body connection established through physical postures. It provides a space for introspection and self-discovery, fostering a deeper understanding of one's inner landscape.

The Intersection of Yoga and Meditation

While yoga and meditation can be practiced independently, they are often intertwined, with many yoga sessions incorporating meditation and vice versa. This integration enhances the overall mind-body experience, creating a synergy that promotes holistic well-being.

The breath, a common focal point in both practices, becomes a bridge connecting the physical and mental aspects of the self. The mindfulness cultivated in meditation seamlessly translates into the mindful movement of yoga, creating a seamless flow of awareness.

Beyond the physical and mental benefits, the mind-body connection fostered by yoga and meditation has implications for emotional and spiritual well-being. Practitioners often report a heightened sense of inner peace, resilience in the face of challenges, and a greater connection to something beyond the self.

The Growing Appeal: Holistic Fitness in Modern Life

The increasing interest in yoga and meditation reflects a broader societal shift towards holistic approaches to health. In a fast-paced world filled with technological distractions and constant stimuli, individuals seek practices that not only keep them physically fit but also nurture their mental and emotional resilience.

The accessibility of yoga and meditation, with classes available in-person and online, caters to diverse preferences and lifestyles. Additionally, the scientific community's growing interest in studying the benefits of these practices has contributed to their mainstream acceptance.

As the evidence supporting the mind-body connection continues to mount, more people are drawn to these ancient practices as tools for maintaining balance in an increasingly complex world.

In conclusion, the rising interest in holistic fitness, driven by the profound mind-body connection, has propelled yoga and meditation into the forefront of wellness practices. Beyond physical exercise, these ancient traditions offer a pathway to mental clarity, emotional well-being, and a deeper understanding of the self. As individuals weave yoga and meditation into their daily lives, the pursuit of holistic health becomes not just a trend but a transformative journey towards a more balanced and harmonious existence.

The Transformative Power Of Yoga And Meditation: A Holistic Approach to Well-being

In a fast-paced world dominated by technology and constant connectivity, the need for holistic well-being has become more apparent than ever. Yoga and meditation, age-old practices rooted in ancient traditions, have emerged as powerful tools to foster a balanced and healthy lifestyle. This article explores the myriad benefits of incorporating yoga and meditation into one's daily routine, shedding light on popular mind-body classes and practices that have gained widespread recognition.

Benefits of Yoga:

1. Physical Well-being:
   Yoga is renowned for its positive impact on physical health. The practice involves a series of

postures, known as asanas, that promote flexibility, strength, and balance. Regular yoga practice can alleviate chronic pain, improve posture, and enhance overall physical fitness.

2. Mental Clarity:

The synchronization of breath and movement in yoga promotes mindfulness, leading to increased mental clarity. This meditative aspect of yoga helps individuals focus on the present moment, reducing stress and anxiety. As a result, practitioners often experience improved cognitive function and emotional well-being.

3. Stress Reduction:

The deep breathing exercises incorporated into yoga trigger the relaxation response in the body, reducing the production of stress hormones. This, in turn, lowers blood pressure and promotes a sense of calm, making yoga an effective tool for stress management.

4. Enhanced Sleep Quality:

Many people struggle with sleep-related issues, and yoga offers a natural remedy. The relaxation techniques practiced in yoga, combined with its ability to calm the nervous system, contribute to better sleep quality. A well-rested body and mind are crucial for overall health.

Benefits of Meditation:

1. **Stress and Anxiety Reduction:**

Meditation is renowned for its ability to calm the mind and reduce stress and anxiety. By cultivating a mindful awareness of thoughts and emotions, individuals can break the cycle of rumination and achieve a more balanced mental state.

2. **Improved Emotional Well-being:**

Regular meditation has been linked to improved emotional regulation and a heightened sense of well-being. It encourages a non-judgmental awareness of one's thoughts and feelings, fostering a positive and compassionate mindset.

3. **Enhanced Concentration and Focus:**

Meditation involves training the mind to focus on the present moment, which can significantly improve concentration and mental clarity. This heightened focus extends beyond meditation sessions, positively impacting various aspects of daily life.

4. **Increased Self-awareness:**

Through introspective practices, meditation allows individuals to explore their inner selves, fostering greater self-awareness. This self-discovery can lead to personal growth, improved decision-making, and a deeper understanding of one's values and priorities.

Popular Mind-Body Classes and Practices:

1. Hatha Yoga:

Hatha yoga is a gentle and accessible form of yoga that focuses on basic postures and breath control. It is an excellent starting point for beginners and provides a solid foundation for other, more advanced yoga practices.

2. Vinyasa Flow:

Vinyasa involves a dynamic sequence of poses synchronized with breath, creating a fluid and rhythmic practice. It offers cardiovascular benefits, enhances flexibility, and promotes a sense of graceful movement.

3. Mindfulness Meditation:

Mindfulness meditation, rooted in Buddhist traditions, emphasizes paying attention to the present moment without judgment. It has gained popularity for its effectiveness in reducing stress, improving focus, and fostering emotional resilience.

4. **Transcendental Meditation**:
   Developed by Maharishi Mahesh Yogi, Transcendental Meditation involves silently repeating a mantra to achieve a state of deep relaxation and heightened awareness. It is known for its simplicity and accessibility.

Finally, Incorporating yoga and meditation into daily life can be a transformative journey toward holistic well-being. These practices offer a myriad of physical, mental, and emotional benefits, making them invaluable tools in the pursuit of a balanced and fulfilling life. Whether through popular mind-body classes or individual practice, embracing these ancient traditions provides a pathway to a healthier, more harmonious existence in our modern world.

CHAPTER 5

OUTDOOR AND ADVENTURE WORKOUTS: Embracing Fitness in Nature

In a world dominated by sedentary lifestyles and indoor activities, outdoor and adventure workouts offer a breath of fresh air – literally. Engaging in physical activity amidst nature not only provides a unique and invigorating experience but also comes with a myriad of health benefits.

Connecting with Nature:
One of the primary appeals of outdoor workouts is the opportunity to connect with nature. Whether it's a trail run through a dense forest, a mountain hike, or a beachside yoga session, these activities allow individuals to escape the hustle and bustle of urban life and immerse themselves in the beauty of the natural world. The sights, sounds, and smells of nature create a multisensory experience that enhances the overall workout.

Variety of Terrain:
Unlike the controlled environment of a gym, outdoor workouts often involve navigating diverse terrains. This variability challenges the body in ways that traditional workouts may not. Running on uneven trails engages stabilizing muscles, hiking uphill builds strength and endurance, and practicing yoga on the beach demands balance on shifting sand. The ever-changing terrain adds an element of unpredictability, keeping both the body and mind stimulated.

Enhanced Mental Well-being:
The mental health benefits of outdoor and adventure workouts are substantial. Spending time in nature has been linked to reduced stress levels, improved mood, and increased overall well-being. The combination of physical activity and natural surroundings triggers the release of endorphins, commonly known as "feel-good" hormones. Additionally, the tranquility of outdoor spaces provides an excellent opportunity for mindfulness and stress relief.

Community and Social Interaction:
Many outdoor workouts are inherently social activities. Group hikes, cycling clubs, and outdoor fitness classes foster a sense of community and camaraderie. Exercising with others not only adds a social dimension but also serves as a motivational factor. The shared experience of conquering a

challenging trail or reaching a summit creates lasting bonds among participants.

Adventurous Spirit:

Adventure workouts go beyond the conventional, encouraging individuals to step out of their comfort zones. From rock climbing to paddleboarding, these activities require a degree of courage and a willingness to embrace the unknown. Overcoming challenges in an outdoor setting not only builds physical strength but also cultivates resilience and a sense of accomplishment.

Low-Cost Fitness:

Outdoor workouts often come with the added benefit of being budget-friendly. Unlike gym memberships or specialized equipment, many outdoor activities require minimal investment. Running shoes, a yoga mat, or a sturdy pair of hiking boots may be the only essentials needed, making fitness accessible to a broader demographic.

Environmental Awareness:

Engaging in outdoor workouts fosters a sense of environmental consciousness. People who spend time in nature are more likely to develop an appreciation for the environment and become advocates for its preservation. This heightened awareness can lead to eco-friendly lifestyle choices and a greater commitment to sustainable practices.

practical tips for outdoor workouts:

1. **Safety First**: Check weather conditions, inform someone about your plans, and carry any necessary safety equipment.
2. **Proper Gear:** Invest in appropriate gear for your chosen activity to ensure comfort and reduce the risk of injury.
3. **Hydration and Nutrition**: Stay hydrated and fuel your body with nutritious snacks, especially during longer outdoor workouts.
4. **Sun Protection**: Use sunscreen, wear appropriate clothing, and protect yourself from the sun's harmful rays.
5. **Respect Nature**: Leave no trace by cleaning up after yourself and respecting wildlife and natural habitats.

In conclusion, outdoor and adventure workouts provide a holistic approach to fitness, combining physical exercise with the rejuvenating effects of nature. Whether you're a seasoned athlete or a fitness enthusiast looking for a change of scenery, venturing outdoors can transform your workout routine into a fulfilling and enriching experience. So, lace up those hiking boots, grab your yoga mat, and embark on a journey to discover the countless benefits of outdoor and adventure workouts.

THE RISE OF OUTDOOR FITNESS ACTIVITIES: EMBRACING NATURE FOR HEALTH AND WELL-being

In recent years, there has been a noticeable shift in fitness trends, with more people opting for outdoor activities to meet their health and wellness goals. The rise of outdoor fitness activities represents a departure from traditional gym workouts and a rediscovery of the benefits that nature can offer in the pursuit of a healthier lifestyle.

Escape from Indoor Confinement:
One of the key factors contributing to the surge in outdoor fitness activities is the desire to break free from the confines of indoor spaces. Modern lifestyles, characterized by sedentary jobs and screen-dominated leisure, have led to a growing disconnect from the natural world. Outdoor workouts provide a welcome escape, allowing individuals to breathe in fresh air, bask in natural sunlight, and enjoy the open spaces that urban environments often lack.

Technology and Outdoor Fitness Apps:

The integration of technology has played a significant role in popularizing outdoor fitness activities. Mobile apps and wearable fitness trackers have empowered individuals to track their progress, set goals, and discover new outdoor workout routines. These apps often include GPS tracking for running and cycling, guided hiking trails, and even virtual personal trainers, creating a seamless blend of technology and nature.

Health Benefits of Outdoor Exercise:

The scientific community has long highlighted the positive impact of outdoor exercise on physical and mental well-being. Exposure to natural light helps regulate circadian rhythms, contributing to better sleep patterns. The increased production of vitamin D from sunlight absorption is crucial for bone health, and the fresh air aids respiratory function. Moreover, outdoor exercise has been linked to reduced stress levels, improved mood, and a lower risk of mental health issues.

Versatility in Outdoor Workouts:

Outdoor fitness activities offer a diverse range of workout options suitable for all fitness levels and preferences. From traditional activities like jogging, hiking, and cycling to more adventurous pursuits such as rock climbing, kayaking, and outdoor yoga, there's something for everyone. The variety in outdoor workouts keeps individuals engaged and motivated, preventing the monotony often associated with indoor routines.

Social Aspect and Community Building:

Participating in outdoor fitness activities often involves a social component, fostering a sense of community among participants. Group runs, outdoor fitness classes, and organized hiking events create opportunities for social interaction and shared experiences. This communal aspect not only enhances the enjoyment of the activity but also provides a support system that can be instrumental in maintaining a regular fitness routine.

Eco-Friendly Fitness:

The rise of outdoor fitness aligns with a growing awareness of environmental sustainability. Unlike traditional gyms with energy-consuming equipment, outdoor workouts have a minimal carbon footprint. Individuals engaging in activities like hiking or cycling reduce their reliance on motorized transportation, promoting eco-friendly modes of commuting while staying fit.

Challenges and Considerations:

While outdoor fitness activities offer numerous benefits, there are challenges to be mindful of. Weather conditions can be unpredictable, necessitating adaptable workout plans. Proper hydration, sun protection, and awareness of one's surroundings are crucial for a safe outdoor fitness experience. Additionally, accessibility to suitable outdoor spaces may vary, requiring individuals to explore and find locations that suit their preferences and fitness goals.

Embracing the Movement:

The rise of outdoor fitness activities is not merely a trend but a cultural shift towards a more holistic and sustainable approach to health and well-being. As more individuals recognize the advantages of combining exercise with the natural world, parks, trails, and outdoor spaces become extensions of the gym, providing diverse and inspiring settings for fitness pursuits.

In conclusion, the rise of outdoor fitness activities signifies a departure from the conventional gym setting, emphasizing the connection between physical health and the great outdoors. Whether it's a solo jog in the park, a group yoga session on the beach, or a challenging mountain hike, outdoor fitness activities empower individuals to reclaim their health while immersing themselves in the beauty of nature. As this movement continues to gain momentum, it not only reshapes the fitness landscape but also redefines our relationship with both exercise and the environment.

INCORPORATING NATURE INTO WORKOUTS

Incorporating nature into workouts offers a refreshing and invigorating approach to physical activity. Instead of confining yourself to a traditional gym setting, you can reap the benefits of exercise while enjoying the natural beauty around you. Here are several ways to seamlessly blend nature with your workouts:

1. **Outdoor Cardiovascular Activities:**
   Embrace the open air by engaging in outdoor cardiovascular exercises. Running or jogging on trails, cycling through scenic routes, or hiking in natural landscapes not only provide an effective workout but also allow you to connect with nature.

2. **Calisthenics in Parks:**
   Many parks are equipped with fitness stations or open spaces suitable for bodyweight exercises. Try incorporating calisthenics routines, such as pull-ups, push-ups, and squats, into your workout regimen. The dynamic surroundings enhance the overall experience.

3. **Yoga and Meditation Outdoors:**
   Take your yoga practice outside and relish in the serenity of nature. Practicing yoga or meditation in

a park or by the beach can deepen your sense of mindfulness, promoting both physical and mental well-being.

4. Water-Based Workouts:

If you're near a body of water, consider integrating water-based exercises. Swimming, paddleboarding, or kayaking not only provide excellent full-body workouts but also allow you to immerse yourself in the calming effects of natural elements.

5. Functional Training in Natural Terrain:

Utilize the varied terrain of outdoor environments for functional training. Incorporate elements like hills, rocks, or sand into your workouts to engage different muscle groups and enhance the overall effectiveness of your routine.

6. Group Fitness in Nature:

Gather a group of friends or join outdoor fitness classes. Many communities offer group workouts in parks or other natural settings, fostering a sense of camaraderie while you collectively benefit from the positive effects of exercising outdoors.

7. Nature-inspired Challenges:

Create fitness challenges inspired by natural elements. For example, design a workout routine that mimics animal movements or incorporate elements of the environment into your exercises, such as using tree branches for balance or elevation changes for intensity.

8. Mindful Walking or Running:

Transform your regular walks or runs into mindful experiences. Pay attention to the sights, sounds, and smells around you, turning your exercise routine into a form of moving meditation that nurtures both your body and mind.

9. **Seasonal Workouts:**

Embrace the changing seasons by adapting your workouts accordingly. In the winter, try cross-country skiing or snowshoeing, while the warmer months may inspire activities like beach volleyball or outdoor circuit training.

10. **Ecotourism Adventures:**

Combine fitness with adventure by exploring ecotourism destinations. Activities like zip-lining, rock climbing, or exploring natural trails not only challenge your physical capabilities but also provide a sense of accomplishment in breathtaking settings.

By integrating nature into your workouts, you not only enhance the physical benefits of exercise but also foster a deeper connection with the world around you, making your fitness journey a holistic and fulfilling experience.

Examples of adventure-based fitness trend

Adventure-based fitness trends have gained significant popularity in recent years, offering individuals a dynamic and engaging way to stay active while exploring their sense of adventure. These trends go beyond conventional workouts, incorporating elements of thrill, exploration, and skill development. Here are some examples of adventure-based fitness trends that have captured the imagination of fitness enthusiasts worldwide:

1. **Obstacle Course Racing (OCR):**

OCR has emerged as a thrilling and challenging adventure-based fitness trend. Events like Spartan Race, Tough Mudder, and Warrior Dash combine running with obstacles such as mud pits, climbing walls, and rope challenges. Participants not only test their physical endurance but also develop mental toughness as they navigate through these demanding courses.

2. **Parkour**:

Parkour, originating from military obstacle course training, has evolved into a popular urban adventure sport. Participants, known as traceurs, use their bodies to move quickly and efficiently through various environments, overcoming obstacles with fluidity and creativity. Parkour fosters strength, agility, and mental focus.

3. Rock Climbing and Bouldering:

Climbing walls and bouldering have become mainstream adventure fitness activities. Indoor climbing gyms provide a controlled environment for beginners, while outdoor rock climbing appeals to those seeking a more authentic and challenging experience. Climbing builds strength, flexibility, and problem-solving skills.

4. Aerial Fitness:

Combining elements of circus arts with fitness, aerial activities like aerial silks, aerial hoop, and pole dancing have gained popularity. These activities require strength, flexibility, and coordination as participants perform acrobatic maneuvers while suspended in the air. Aerial fitness provides a unique and empowering workout experience.

5. Adventure Racing:

Adventure races, such as the Eco-Challenge and Raid Gauloises, combine multiple disciplines like running, mountain biking, kayaking, and navigation in a challenging, often wilderness setting. Teams navigate through a series of checkpoints, promoting teamwork, strategy, and resilience in the face of unpredictable conditions.

6. **Surfing Workouts:**

Surfing has inspired fitness programs that mimic the movements and demands of riding waves. Surf-inspired workouts often incorporate balance training, core exercises, and cardiovascular conditioning. These workouts not only improve surfing skills but also provide a fun and effective way to stay in shape.

7. **Wilderness Survival Workshops**:

Wilderness survival workshops blend fitness with essential outdoor skills. Participants learn to navigate and survive in the wild, incorporating activities like fire-building, shelter construction, and foraging. These workshops enhance physical fitness while imparting valuable survival knowledge.

8. **Adventure Yoga Retreats:**

Adventure yoga retreats combine the tranquility of yoga with outdoor exploration. Participants engage in yoga sessions amidst natural landscapes, incorporating activities like hiking, kayaking, or zip-lining. These retreats offer a holistic approach to fitness, combining mindful practices with physical activity.

9. **Stand-Up Paddleboard (SUP) Fitness:**

SUP fitness involves performing exercises on a paddleboard, adding an element of balance and stability to traditional workouts. Whether it's yoga, strength training, or cardio exercises, SUP fitness provides a unique and serene way to stay fit on the water.

10. **Mountain Biking Adventures:**

Mountain biking has evolved into more than just a sport; it's a thrilling adventure that combines cardiovascular exercise with technical skill. Trail riding in diverse terrains challenges riders physically and mentally, making it an exhilarating way to stay fit while exploring nature.

These adventure-based fitness trends cater to individuals seeking excitement and variety in their workouts. By embracing these activities, fitness enthusiasts not only enhance their physical well-being but also experience a sense of accomplishment and connection with the outdoors. As these trends continue to evolve, the fusion of fitness and adventure is likely to inspire even more innovative and exciting ways for people to stay active.

CHAPTER 6

GROUP FITNESS DYNAMICS

Group fitness dynamics involve the interplay of various factors within a fitness class setting, creating a unique environment that influences participants' experiences and outcomes. These dynamics encompass social, motivational, and instructional elements that contribute to the overall effectiveness and enjoyment of group fitness activities.

1. **Social Interaction:**

Group fitness provides a social platform where individuals with similar health and fitness goals come together. The sense of community fosters motivation and accountability, as participants often form connections and build supportive relationships. Social dynamics play a crucial role in sustaining long-term adherence to exercise routines, as the camaraderie within the group can enhance the overall fitness experience.

2. **Motivational Factors:**

The motivational aspect of group fitness is multifaceted. Firstly, the presence of others creates a positive peer pressure that encourages individuals to push their limits and strive for improvement. Group settings often involve energetic instructors who serve as motivators, guiding participants through workouts and inspiring them to overcome challenges. Additionally, the collective energy of a group can elevate motivation, making participants more likely to stay committed to their fitness journey.

3. **Instruction and Guidance:**

Effective instruction is fundamental to group fitness dynamics. Instructors play a pivotal role in creating a positive and inclusive atmosphere, ensuring that participants feel comfortable and capable. Clear communication, proper demonstration, and personalized guidance contribute to a supportive learning environment. The instructor's ability to adapt to diverse fitness levels within the group enhances the overall experience and maximizes the benefits for each participant.

4. **Diversity of Workouts:**

Group fitness classes often offer a diverse range of workouts, catering to various preferences and fitness levels. This diversity not only prevents monotony but also allows participants to explore different exercise modalities, promoting overall fitness and preventing plateaus. The dynamic nature of group workouts, whether it's high-intensity interval training (HIIT), dance-based classes, or strength training, contributes to a holistic approach to health and wellness.

5. **Psychological Benefits:**

Beyond the physical aspects, group fitness dynamics impact mental and emotional well-being. The collective energy and positive reinforcement within a group can alleviate stress, reduce anxiety, and enhance mood. The shared sense of achievement after completing a challenging workout fosters a positive mindset and contributes to the overall mental health of participants.

6. **Accountability and Consistency:**

The group setting inherently fosters a sense of accountability. Knowing that others are expecting your presence can be a powerful motivator to adhere to a regular exercise routine. Consistency, in turn, is key to achieving fitness goals, and the group dynamics create a structured environment that supports ongoing commitment.

In conclusion, group fitness dynamics encompass the intricate interplay of social, motivational, instructional, and psychological elements. This holistic approach contributes to a positive and enriching fitness experience, making group fitness an effective and enjoyable way for individuals to pursue their health and wellness goals.

ANALYSIS OF GROUP FITNESS CLASSES:

Group fitness classes undergo comprehensive evaluation to assess their effectiveness, appeal, and overall impact on participants. This analysis involves a multidimensional approach, considering various aspects that contribute to the success and sustainability of these classes.

1. Program Design and Structure:

The foundation of a group fitness class lies in its program design. An effective analysis begins by scrutinizing the structure of the class, including the progression of exercises, intensity levels, and duration. A well-designed program should cater to diverse fitness levels within the group, providing modifications for beginners and challenges for advanced participants.

2. **Instructor Competence:**

The competence and expertise of the instructor significantly influence the success of a group fitness class. Analysis involves evaluating the instructor's ability to provide clear instructions, offer modifications, and create a motivational and inclusive atmosphere. Instructor knowledge about anatomy, exercise physiology, and proper form is crucial for ensuring participant safety and maximizing the benefits of the workout.

3. **Participant Engagement:**

The level of participant engagement serves as a key metric in the analysis of group fitness classes. Observing whether participants are actively involved, motivated, and enjoying the class helps gauge its effectiveness. Interaction within the group, responsiveness to the instructor's cues, and the overall energy of the class contribute to a positive environment.

4. **Variety and Innovation:**

Successful group fitness classes incorporate variety and innovation to prevent monotony. Analysis considers whether the class offers a diverse range of exercises, utilizes different training modalities, and introduces new elements periodically. This ensures sustained interest among participants and prevents plateaus in fitness progression.

5. **Inclusivity and Adaptability:**

Inclusivity is a critical aspect of group fitness analysis. The class should be designed to accommodate participants with varying fitness levels, abilities, and limitations. Analyzing how well the class adapts to different needs ensures that it remains accessible and welcoming to a diverse audience.

6. **Monitoring Intensity Levels:**

The intensity of a group fitness class should align with the stated goals and the fitness levels of the participants. Analysis involves monitoring heart rate zones, perceived exertion, and the overall metabolic demand of the workout. This ensures that the class delivers the intended physiological benefits while minimizing the risk of overtraining or injury.

7. **Feedback and Assessment:**

Collecting feedback from participants and conducting periodic assessments are integral components of group fitness class analysis. Surveys, focus group discussions, and individual assessments help identify strengths and areas for improvement. Regular feedback loops facilitate continuous refinement of the class to meet the evolving needs and preferences of participants.

8. **Community Building:**

Group fitness classes often contribute to community building within fitness facilities. Analysis explores the social dynamics, camaraderie, and sense of belonging that the class fosters. Assessing the community aspect helps gauge the long-term adherence of participants and their overall satisfaction with the class experience.

9. **Technology Integration:**

In the modern fitness landscape, technology plays a significant role. Analysis includes the integration of technology, such as heart rate monitoring, virtual platforms, or interactive elements, to enhance the overall class experience and provide additional data for participants and instructors.

In conclusion, a thorough analysis of group fitness classes involves examining program design, instructor competence, participant engagement, variety, inclusivity, intensity levels, feedback mechanisms, community building, and technology integration. This holistic evaluation ensures that group fitness classes remain dynamic, effective, and appealing to a diverse audience, contributing to the overall success of fitness programs.

SOCIAL AND MOTIVATIONAL ASPECTS IN FITNESS:

1. Community Building:

One of the key social aspects of fitness is the sense of community it fosters. Group fitness classes, team sports, or workout groups create a supportive environment where individuals share common goals. This sense of belonging and camaraderie not only enhances the overall experience but also contributes to long-term adherence to exercise routines.

2. Positive Peer Pressure:

The social setting of fitness activities introduces an element of positive peer pressure. Working out alongside others can motivate individuals to push their limits, strive for improvement, and stay consistent with their fitness routines. Observing the dedication and progress of fellow participants often serves as a powerful motivator.

3. Instructor-Participant Relationship:

The relationship between fitness instructors and participants plays a crucial role in the motivational aspect. Instructors who are not only knowledgeable but also encouraging and approachable create a positive and motivating atmosphere. Their ability to provide constructive feedback and support contributes to the overall satisfaction and commitment of participants.

4. **Group Energy and Dynamics:**

The energy generated within a group setting is contagious. The collective enthusiasm, shared effort, and synchronized movements create a dynamic environment that can significantly enhance motivation. This group energy often leads to increased intensity and effort, resulting in more effective workouts.

5. **Social Accountability:**

The social aspect of fitness introduces a form of accountability. When individuals commit to group activities or workout partners, they feel a sense of responsibility not only to themselves but also to the group. This accountability can be a powerful motivator, encouraging individuals to show up consistently and put in their best effort.

6. **Goal Sharing and Celebration:**

Setting and achieving fitness goals become more meaningful when shared with others. In a social fitness setting, participants often celebrate milestones together, fostering a sense of achievement and motivation to set new goals. This shared journey creates a positive feedback loop that propels individuals forward in their fitness endeavors.

7. Variety and Social Interaction:

Social aspects often contribute to the variety of workouts. Group fitness classes or team sports introduce diversity in exercises and activities, making workouts more enjoyable. Additionally, the social interaction during these activities can turn a routine workout into a social event, enhancing the overall experience.

8. Mental and Emotional Support:

Beyond the physical benefits, the social aspect of fitness provides mental and emotional support. Participants often form connections, share experiences, and provide encouragement during challenging times. This support network contributes to stress reduction, improved mood, and a positive mindset.

9. Competitive Motivation:

In certain fitness settings, friendly competition can be a motivating factor. Whether it's competing with others or oneself, the social environment introduces a healthy level of competition that can drive individuals to improve their performance and achieve better results.

10. Flexibility and Adaptability:

Social and motivational aspects in fitness contribute to adaptability. Group dynamics allow for flexible approaches to workouts, accommodating different fitness levels and preferences. This adaptability ensures that individuals find motivation in a way that suits their unique needs and circumstances.

In conclusion, the social and motivational aspects of fitness are integral components that go beyond the physical benefits. Building a sense of community, fostering positive peer pressure, nurturing instructor-participant relationships, harnessing group energy, and providing mental and emotional support all contribute to creating a motivating and enjoyable fitness experience. These aspects play a crucial role in long-term adherence to healthy lifestyles and overall well-being.

EXAMPLE OF TRENDING GROUP WORKOUTS:

Group workouts have evolved with fitness trends, offering diverse and dynamic experiences that cater to varying preferences. Here are some examples of trending group workouts that have gained popularity in recent times:

1. **High-Intensity Interval Training (HIIT) Classes**:
HIIT continues to be a dominant trend in group fitness. These classes involve short bursts of intense exercise followed by brief rest periods. The fast-paced, efficient nature of HIIT appeals to those looking for effective workouts in a time-efficient manner.

2. **Boutique Fitness Classes:**
Boutique fitness studios specializing in specific workout modalities have gained popularity. Examples include cycling classes (such as SoulCycle), barre workouts (like Pure Barre), and specialized strength training sessions. These studios often provide a unique and immersive experience.

3. **Dance Fitness:**
Dance-based group workouts, like Zumba or dance cardio classes, have become widely popular. These sessions combine energetic dance routines with music, making them not only effective for fitness but also enjoyable and engaging.

4. **Functional Fitness Groups:**
Functional fitness emphasizes movements that mimic real-life activities. Group classes incorporating functional exercises, such as kettlebell workouts, TRX training, and bodyweight exercises, focus on building strength and flexibility.

5. **Outdoor Boot Camps:**

Fitness boot camps conducted outdoors have gained traction. These classes often blend cardiovascular exercises with strength training in an outdoor setting, providing a refreshing alternative to traditional gym workouts.

6. **Mind-Body Classes:**

Classes that integrate mindfulness and body awareness, such as yoga and Pilates, continue to be popular. These workouts not only improve flexibility and strength but also promote mental well-being and stress reduction.

7. **Rowing Classes:**

Indoor rowing classes have emerged as a full-body, low-impact workout option. These classes often include rowing intervals combined with strength training, providing a unique and effective group fitness experience.

8. **CrossFit**:

CrossFit remains a notable trend in group fitness, combining elements of weightlifting, cardio, and gymnastics. CrossFit classes are known for their intensity, variety, and sense of community.

9. **Virtual Fitness Classes:**

With the rise of technology, virtual group fitness classes have become popular. Platforms offering live or on-demand group workouts allow participants to join sessions from the comfort of their homes, providing flexibility and accessibility.

10. **Boxing and Martial Arts Workouts:**

Group workouts incorporating elements of boxing or martial arts, such as kickboxing or mixed martial arts (MMA) classes, have gained popularity. These classes often blend cardiovascular training with strength and agility exercises.

11. **Circuit Training:**

Circuit training involves moving through a series of different exercises with minimal rest between them. Group circuit training classes offer a dynamic and time-efficient way to work on various fitness components.

12. **Aerial Fitness:**

Aerial workouts, such as aerial yoga or aerial silks, provide a unique and challenging group fitness experience. These classes often focus on flexibility, core strength, and body awareness.

13. **Aquatic Fitness Classes:**

Water-based group workouts, including aqua aerobics and water cycling, offer a low-impact yet effective way to improve cardiovascular fitness and strength.

CHAPTER 7

Nutrition and fitness integration

Nutrition and fitness integration is a holistic approach that combines dietary habits with physical activity to promote overall health and well-being. This synergistic relationship between nutrition and fitness is crucial for achieving optimal results in terms of weight management, muscle development, and overall vitality.

1. **Fueling the Body:**
   - Proper nutrition serves as the foundation for any successful fitness regimen. It provides the body with the necessary fuel to perform optimally during exercise and aids in recovery afterward.
   - Macronutrients including carbohydrates, proteins, and lipids each perform a unique role. Carbohydrates are essential for energy, proteins for muscle repair and growth, and fats for overall health and hormonal balance.

2. **Pre-Workout Nutrition:**
   - Consuming a balanced meal or snack before a workout is vital. It ensures that the body has enough energy to sustain the physical activity and helps prevent muscle breakdown.

- A combination of carbohydrates and proteins is often recommended for pre-workout nutrition. This could include a banana with peanut butter or Greek yogurt with berries.

3. **Hydration**:

- Adequate hydration is a cornerstone of both nutrition and fitness. Water is essential for digestion, nutrient absorption, and temperature regulation during exercise.
- Maintaining proper fluid balance is critical for preventing dehydration, which can negatively impact exercise performance and recovery.

4. **Post-Workout Nutrition:**

- After a workout, the body requires nutrients to replenish glycogen stores and support muscle recovery. A post-workout meal or snack should include a balance of carbohydrates and proteins.
- Examples include a protein shake, a chicken and vegetable stir-fry with quinoa, or a yogurt parfait with fruit and granola.

5. **Weight Management:**

- Integrating nutrition and fitness is fundamental for weight management. A combination of a healthy, balanced diet and regular exercise helps in achieving and maintaining a healthy weight.
- Caloric intake should align with individual goals, whether it's weight loss, maintenance, or muscle gain.

6. **Individualized Approaches:**
   - Every person is unique, and nutritional needs vary based on factors such as age, gender, metabolism, and fitness goals. Tailoring both nutrition and fitness plans to individual requirements is key for success.
   - Consulting with a registered dietitian or nutritionist, as well as a fitness professional, can help in developing personalized strategies.

7. **Long-Term Health Benefits**:
   - The integration of nutrition and fitness goes beyond immediate physical goals; it contributes to long-term health. Regular physical activity and a balanced diet reduce the risk of chronic diseases such as heart disease, diabetes, and obesity.
   - Establishing healthy habits early in life and maintaining them throughout the lifespan is essential for overall well-being.

In conclusion, nutrition and fitness integration is a dynamic and interconnected approach that maximizes the benefits of both aspects for a healthier and more fulfilling lifestyle. It's not just about what you eat or how you exercise; it's about combining these elements in a way that supports your unique health and fitness goals.

IMPORTANCE OF NUTRITION IN ACHIEVING FITNESS GOALS

The importance of nutrition in achieving fitness goals cannot be overstated; it is a cornerstone that significantly influences the effectiveness of any fitness regimen. Nutrition plays a pivotal role in various aspects of physical well-being, ranging from energy levels and performance to recovery and overall health.

1. Energy Source:

- Proper nutrition provides the body with the necessary fuel for physical activity. Carbohydrates are the primary source of energy, and they are crucial for sustained endurance during workouts.
- Insufficient carbohydrate intake can lead to fatigue, negatively impacting exercise performance and hindering the ability to achieve fitness goals.

2. Muscle Repair and Growth:

- Protein, one of the essential macronutrients, is paramount for muscle repair and growth. Engaging in regular exercise places stress on muscles, and adequate protein intake supports their recovery and development.
- Athletes and individuals aiming for muscle hypertrophy often require a higher protein intake to optimize these processes.

3. **Nutrient Timing:**
   - The timing of nutrient intake is critical for maximizing fitness outcomes. Pre-workout nutrition ensures the body has sufficient energy reserves, while post-workout nutrition supports recovery and muscle synthesis.
   - Consuming a balanced meal or snack with the right macronutrient composition before and after exercise aids in achieving optimal performance and effective recovery.

4. Metabolism and Weight Management:
   - Nutrition influences metabolism, the body's process of converting food into energy. A well-balanced diet helps regulate metabolism, supporting weight management goals.
   - Eating the right types and amounts of nutrients contributes to maintaining a healthy body composition, whether the goal is weight loss, muscle gain, or overall fitness.

5. **Hydration and Exercise Performance:**
   - Proper hydration is integral to achieving fitness goals. Dehydration can lead to decreased exercise performance, impaired recovery, and increased risk of injury.
   - Water is essential for various physiological processes, including nutrient transport, temperature regulation, and joint lubrication, all of which contribute to optimal exercise performance.

6. **Mental Focus and Endurance:**
   - Nutrient-rich foods not only fuel the body but also support cognitive function. Adequate nutrition positively impacts mental focus and concentration during workouts.
   - Complex carbohydrates, found in foods like whole grains and fruits, provide a steady release of energy, sustaining endurance and preventing mental fatigue during prolonged exercise.

7. **Overall Health and Longevity:**
   - Nutrition is a fundamental component of overall health and longevity. A well-rounded, nutrient-dense diet supports immune function, reduces the risk of chronic diseases, and enhances the body's ability to recover from physical stress.
   - Adopting healthy eating habits contributes to sustained well-being, allowing individuals to engage in consistent and effective exercise over the long term.

In summary, achieving fitness goals requires a harmonious integration of nutrition and exercise. Proper nutrition not only enhances physical performance but also supports recovery, muscle development, and overall health. Recognizing the symbiotic relationship between nutrition and fitness is essential for individuals seeking to optimize their training and reach their fitness objectives.

TRENDS IN FITNESS-ORIENTED DIETS:

1. Plant-Based Diets:
   - The rise of plant-based diets, such as vegetarianism and veganism, reflects a growing interest in sustainable and ethical eating. Plant-based diets emphasize fruits, vegetables, grains, and legumes, providing essential nutrients for fitness enthusiasts.

2. Keto Diet:
   - The ketogenic diet, characterized by low-carbohydrate and high-fat intake, has gained popularity for its potential to promote weight loss and improve endurance. The body burns fat for energy when it enters a state of ketosis, which is encouraged by it..

3. Intermittent Fasting:
   - Intermittent fasting occurs between eating and fasting intervals.
. This trend is embraced for its potential benefits in weight management, improved metabolism, and enhanced fat burning during fasting periods.

4. Protein-First Approach:
   - Many fitness-oriented diets emphasize a higher protein intake to support muscle development and recovery. Protein-centric diets may include lean

meats, dairy, plant-based protein sources, and supplements to meet increased protein needs.

5. **Personalized Nutrition:**

   - Tailoring diets to individual needs based on factors like body type, metabolism, and fitness goals is a growing trend. Personalized nutrition involves using genetic information or individual preferences to create customized eating plans.

6. **Functional Foods and Supplements:**

   - The incorporation of functional foods and targeted supplements is on the rise. Fitness enthusiasts are exploring foods with added health benefits, such as fortified snacks and beverages, as well as supplements like collagen, omega-3 fatty acids, and adaptogens.

7. **Mindful Eating:**

   - - When consuming food, mindful eating involves being mindful about the present moment while consuming food. This trend encourages individuals to savor each bite, be aware of hunger and fullness cues, and make conscious food choices that align with fitness goals.

TIPS FOR COMBINING NUTRITION AND EXERCISE EFFECTIVELY:

1. Set Realistic Goals:

- Clearly define fitness goals and align nutritional choices with those objectives. Whether it's weight loss, muscle gain, or overall well-being, understanding specific goals is crucial for effective integration.

2. Balance Macronutrients:

- Ensure a balanced intake of carbohydrates, proteins, and fats to support energy needs, muscle recovery, and overall health. The proportion of macronutrients can be adjusted based on individual preferences and fitness goals.

3. Timing Matters:

- Pay attention to nutrient timing. Consume a balanced meal or snack before workouts for energy and afterward to support recovery. Timing nutrient intake optimally enhances exercise performance and aids in achieving fitness goals.

4. Stay Hydrated:

- Adequate hydration is essential for optimal exercise performance and recovery. Water is crucial for nutrient transport, temperature regulation, and joint lubrication. Throughout the day, drink more water, especially when working out.

5. **Variety in Diet:**
   - Embrace a diverse and nutrient-rich diet. Include a variety of fruits, vegetables, whole grains, lean proteins, and healthy fats to ensure a broad spectrum of essential nutrients for overall health and fitness.

6. **Listen to Your Body:**
   - Pay attention to hunger and fullness cues. Listen to your body's signals, and avoid restrictive eating habits. Eating in tune with your body's needs fosters a healthy relationship with food and supports sustainable fitness practices.

7. **Consult Professionals:**
   - Seek guidance from certified nutritionists, dietitians, and fitness professionals. They can provide personalized advice based on individual needs, ensuring a safe and effective approach to combining nutrition and exercise.

Incorporating these trends and tips into one's lifestyle can contribute to a well-rounded and effective approach to fitness-oriented diets, promoting not only physical health but also overall well-being.

CHAPTER 8

RECOVERY AND WELLNESS TECHNIQUES

Recovery and wellness techniques encompass a variety of approaches aimed at promoting physical, mental, and emotional well-being. These strategies are designed to help individuals bounce back from stress, illness, or challenging situations, fostering a holistic sense of health. Here are some key aspects of recovery and wellness techniques:

1. Physical Well-being:

- **Exercise**: Regular physical activity is crucial for overall well-being. It not only enhances cardiovascular health but also releases endorphins, reducing stress and promoting a positive mood.

- **Nutrition**: A balanced and nutritious diet provides the body with essential nutrients, contributing to physical recovery and maintaining optimal health.

2. Mental Health:

- **Mindfulness and Meditation:** These practices involve focusing on the present moment, reducing stress and promoting mental clarity. Mindfulness and meditation have been linked to improved cognitive function and emotional well-being.
- **Therapy and Counseling:** Professional psychological support can aid in overcoming challenges, managing stress, and fostering emotional resilience.

3. Rest and Sleep:

- **Quality Sleep**: Adequate and quality sleep is fundamental for recovery. It allows the body to repair itself, supports cognitive function, and contributes to emotional balance.

4. Social Connection:

- **Social Support:** Building and maintaining strong social connections can provide a vital support system during challenging times. It offers emotional support, reduces feelings of isolation, and contributes to overall well-being.

5. Holistic Approaches:

- **Yoga**: Combining physical postures, breath control, and meditation, yoga promotes flexibility, strength, and mental calmness.
- **Acupuncture and Massage:** These alternative therapies can contribute to physical and mental relaxation, easing tension and promoting overall wellness.

6. Self-Care Practices:

- **Hobbies and Recreation:** Engaging in activities that bring joy and relaxation, such as hobbies and recreational pursuits, is essential for maintaining a balanced and fulfilling life.
- **Digital Detox:** Taking breaks from constant connectivity and screen time can improve mental well-being and reduce stress.

7. Goal Setting and Time Management:

- **Setting Realistic Goals:** Establishing achievable objectives fosters a sense of accomplishment and motivation.
- **Effective Time Management:** Organizing and prioritizing tasks can reduce stress and improve productivity, contributing to overall well-being.

8. **Resilience Building**:

   - **Coping Strategies**: Developing effective coping mechanisms helps individuals navigate challenges and bounce back from setbacks.
   - **Learning from Adversity**: Viewing challenges as opportunities for growth can enhance resilience and promote a positive mindset.

Incorporating a combination of these recovery and wellness techniques into one's lifestyle can contribute to a healthier, more balanced, and resilient life. It's important to recognize that individual preferences may vary, and finding the right combination of practices is a personal journey toward well-being.

FOCUS ON RECOVERY AS AN ESSENTIAL PART OF FITNESS:

In the realm of fitness, there has been a paradigm shift in recent years, acknowledging that recovery is not merely a passive phase but an active and crucial component of any effective training regimen. Fitness enthusiasts and athletes alike are recognizing that achieving optimal performance goes beyond intense workouts – it involves a holistic approach that incorporates adequate recovery strategies. Here's an in-depth exploration of why focusing on recovery is considered an indispensable aspect of fitness:

1. Muscle Repair and Growth:

- **Importance of Rest Days**: Intense exercise induces microscopic damage to muscle fibers. Adequate rest and recovery days allow these fibers to repair and grow, contributing to strength and muscle development.
- **Sleep Quality**: During sleep, the body releases growth hormone, essential for muscle repair. Poor sleep patterns can hinder this process, emphasizing the link between recovery and sleep.

2. Injury Prevention:

- **Overtraining Risks**: Continuous, high-intensity training without proper recovery increases the risk of overtraining. Overtraining can lead to fatigue, compromised immune function, and a higher susceptibility to injuries.
- **Active Recovery**: Incorporating light exercises, stretching, or activities like yoga on rest days can enhance blood circulation, alleviate muscle stiffness, and reduce the risk of injuries.

3. Optimizing Performance:

- **Reducing Fatigue:** Regular recovery practices, such as foam rolling and massage, can alleviate muscle tightness and reduce overall fatigue. This can enhance an individual's ability to perform at their best during workouts.

- **Nutrient Timing:** Consuming the right nutrients post-exercise supports glycogen replenishment and muscle recovery, optimizing the body for subsequent training sessions.

4. Balancing Stress Hormones:

- **Cortisol Management**: Intense exercise elevates cortisol levels, the body's stress hormone. Chronic elevation can lead to muscle breakdown and hinder recovery. Adequate rest and stress-reducing activities help manage cortisol levels.

- **Mind-Body Connection**: Techniques like meditation and mindfulness not only contribute to mental well-being but also aid in balancing stress hormones, promoting a healthier physiological environment for recovery.

5. Joint and Connective Tissue Health:
- **Impact of High-Intensity Exercise:**
Rigorous training can stress joints and connective tissues. Adequate recovery allows these structures

to adapt and strengthen, reducing the risk of
overuse injuries.

   - **Hydration and Nutrition:** Proper hydration
and nutrition support joint health and the body's
ability to repair connective tissues.

6. Psychological Well-being:

   - **Burnout Prevention**: Continuous, strenuous
training without sufficient recovery can lead to
burnout. Incorporating rest days and varied
activities helps prevent mental fatigue and
maintains a positive attitude towards fitness.

   - **Enjoyment and Longevity:** Emphasizing the
enjoyment of physical activity and recognizing the
long-term nature of fitness goals contribute to a
sustainable and balanced approach.

7. Individualization of Recovery Strategies:

   - **Tailoring Recovery to Individual Needs**:
Every individual responds differently to exercise
and recovery strategies. Personalizing recovery
techniques, such as ice baths, compression
therapy, or specific stretches, can optimize results.

In summary, acknowledging recovery as an
essential part of fitness is fundamental for
achieving long-term health and performance goals.
It's not about the quantity of training alone but the
quality of recovery that ultimately determines the
success of a fitness journey. Balancing intensity

with proper rest, nutrition, and overall well-being creates a foundation for sustainable fitness progress.

OVERVIEW OF RECOVERY METHODS:

Recovery methods play a pivotal role in optimizing physical performance, preventing injuries, and supporting overall well-being. Here is an extensive overview of various recovery techniques that individuals can incorporate into their fitness routines:

1. **Active Recovery:**
   - **Light Exercise**: Engaging in low-intensity activities like walking, swimming, or cycling on rest days promotes blood flow, aiding in the removal of metabolic waste products and reducing muscle stiffness.

2. **Stretching and Flexibility Training:**
   - **Stretching**: Holding stretches for specific muscle groups improves flexibility and reduces muscle tension. Incorporating dynamic stretching before workouts enhances joint mobility and prepares the body for exercise.

3. **Foam Rolling and Self-Myofascial Release:**

   - **Foam Rollers:** Applying pressure to specific muscle areas using foam rollers helps release tension, improve flexibility, and alleviate muscle soreness by breaking down adhesions in the fascia.

4. **Massage Therapy**:

   - **Professional Massage**: Regular massages can enhance blood circulation, reduce muscle tightness, and promote relaxation. Different massage techniques target specific muscle groups and aid in overall recovery.

5. **Compression Therapy:**

   - **Compression Garments**: These garments apply pressure to limbs, promoting blood flow and reducing inflammation. Compression therapy is often used to speed up recovery after intense workouts or competitions.

6. **Cold Therapy**:

   - **Ice Baths:** Immersing the body in cold water reduces inflammation, minimizes muscle soreness, and enhances recovery. Cold therapy can also be applied through ice packs or cryotherapy chambers.

7. **Heat Therapy**:

   - **Saunas and Hot Baths:** Heat therapy increases blood flow, relaxes muscles, and promotes the elimination of toxins. Saunas and hot baths can aid in muscle recovery and provide a relaxing experience.

8. **Nutrition and Hydration:**
   - **Post-Exercise Nutrition**: Consuming a balanced combination of carbohydrates and protein within the post-exercise window supports muscle glycogen replenishment and protein synthesis.
   - **Hydration**: Staying adequately hydrated is essential for overall health and aids in the efficient transport of nutrients to cells.

9. **Sleep and Rest:**
   - **Quality Sleep**: Sleep is a crucial component of recovery, allowing the body to repair tissues, release growth hormone, and consolidate memories. Lack of sleep can negatively impact cognitive function, mood, and physical performance.

10. **Mindfulness and Relaxation Techniques**:
   - **Meditation and Yoga**: Mindfulness practices reduce stress, improve focus, and contribute to overall well-being. Yoga combines physical postures with breath control and meditation, promoting flexibility and relaxation.

11. **Electrotherapy**:
   - **Electrical Muscle Stimulation (EMS):** EMS devices deliver electrical impulses to muscles,

promoting blood circulation and aiding in recovery. These devices are often used for muscle rehabilitation and soreness relief.

12. Periodization and Deload Weeks:
- **Structured Training Cycles**: Incorporating planned periods of reduced intensity, known as deload weeks, helps prevent overtraining and allows the body to recover fully before progressing to more intense workouts.

IMPORTANCE OF REST AND SLEEP IN THE FITNESS Journey:

Rest and sleep are often underestimated components of a successful fitness journey. They are essential for both physical and mental recovery, playing a crucial role in achieving fitness goals. Here's an in-depth look at why rest and sleep are integral:

1. **Muscle Repair and Growth**:
- **During Sleep**: Growth hormone, essential for muscle repair and growth, is predominantly released during deep sleep stages. Quality sleep supports the body's ability to recover from the stresses of exercise.

2. **Hormonal Balance:**
   - **Cortisol Regulation:** Adequate sleep helps regulate cortisol levels, preventing the excessive release of this stress hormone associated with muscle breakdown and impaired recovery.

3. **Energy Restoration:**
   - **Glycogen Replenishment:** During sleep, the body replenishes glycogen stores in muscles and the liver. This process ensures energy availability for subsequent workouts.

4. **Immune System Support:**
   - **During Rest:** The immune system is actively engaged in repair and defense mechanisms. Consistent, quality sleep supports immune function, reducing the risk of illness and enhancing overall well-being.

5. **Cognitive Function:**
   - **Memory Consolidation:** Sleep is crucial for consolidating memories, including motor skills and information learned during workouts. It positively impacts cognitive function, focus, and decision-making.

6. **Injury Prevention:**
   - **Reducing Fatigue:** Inadequate sleep increases fatigue, impairing coordination and reaction time.

This fatigue can contribute to an elevated risk of injuries during physical activities.

7. **Mood and Mental Health:**

- **Stress Reduction**: Quality sleep contributes to stress reduction, positively impacting mental health. Chronic sleep deprivation is associated with increased stress levels and mood disturbances.

8. **Optimizing Performance**:

- **Reaction** Time: Adequate sleep improves reaction time and alertness, optimizing performance during workouts or athletic activities.

9. **Recovery from Mental Fatigue:**

- **Cognitive Restoration**: Sleep serves as a period of cognitive restoration, allowing the brain to recover from the mental fatigue associated with daily activities and intense training.

10. **Individual Sleep Needs**:

Varied Sleep Requirements: Individual sleep needs vary, but most adults generally require 7-9 hours of quality sleep per night. Understanding and meeting one's sleep needs are vital for long-term health and fitness.

In conclusion, recognizing the significance of rest and sleep as integral components of the fitness journey is crucial for achieving sustainable results. Balancing challenging workouts with adequate recovery, including quality sleep, supports overall well-being and ensures that the body is prepared for the demands of an active lifestyle.

CHAPTER 9

VIRTUAL FITNESS EXPERIENCES

Virtual fitness experiences have gained significant popularity in recent years, offering individuals a convenient and engaging way to stay active and healthy. These experiences leverage technology to bring fitness routines, classes, and personal training sessions directly to users' screens, allowing them to participate from the comfort of their homes or any location with an internet connection.

One of the key advantages of virtual fitness experiences is accessibility. People no longer need to commute to a gym or a fitness studio; instead, they can access a wide variety of workouts through online platforms. This accessibility is particularly beneficial for individuals with busy schedules, those in remote areas, or those who prefer the privacy of home workouts.

These virtual experiences often include live-streamed classes, on-demand workout videos, and interactive fitness apps. Live classes provide real-time interaction with instructors and a sense of community as participants from around the world join in simultaneously. On-demand videos, on the other hand, offer flexibility, allowing users to choose workouts that suit their preferences and schedules.

In addition to traditional workouts, virtual fitness experiences often incorporate innovative technologies to enhance engagement. Virtual reality (VR) and augmented reality (AR) are examples of technologies that can transform the fitness landscape. VR can transport users to immersive environments, making workouts more enjoyable and motivating. AR, on the other hand, can overlay digital information on the real world, providing guidance and feedback during exercises.

Personalization is another key aspect of virtual fitness experiences. Many platforms use algorithms to tailor workouts based on users' fitness levels, goals, and preferences. This personalized approach can make the fitness journey more effective and enjoyable, as individuals receive recommendations that align with their specific needs.

Moreover, virtual fitness experiences have become a bridge to connect fitness professionals with a global audience. Trainers and instructors can reach clients beyond geographical constraints, expanding their reach and impact. This not only benefits fitness professionals but also provides users with access to a diverse range of expertise and training styles.

Despite these advantages, there are challenges associated with virtual fitness experiences. Some individuals may struggle with motivation or find it challenging to maintain a consistent routine without the physical presence of a gym or class. Technical issues, such as internet connectivity problems or device compatibility issues, can also hinder the overall experience.

In conclusion, virtual fitness experiences represent a transformative trend in the fitness industry, offering accessibility, convenience, and innovation. As technology continues to advance, we can expect further developments in virtual reality, augmented reality, and personalized fitness solutions, providing individuals with even more engaging and effective ways to pursue a healthy and active lifestyle.

IMPACT OF TECHNOLOGY ON VIRTUAL FITNESS

The impact of technology on virtual fitness has been profound, revolutionizing the way individuals approach and engage in their fitness routines. Several key aspects highlight the transformative influence of technology in this domain.

1. **Accessibility and Convenience**:
   Fitness is now more accessible than before due to technological advances. Virtual fitness platforms allow users to access a wide range of workouts, classes, and training sessions from the convenience of their homes. This accessibility eliminates barriers such as distance, time constraints, and the need for specialized equipment, making it easier for people to integrate regular exercise into their lives.

2. **Interactive Workouts**:
   Virtual fitness experiences leverage interactive technologies to create engaging workouts. Live-streamed classes enable real-time interaction between instructors and participants, fostering a sense of community. This interactivity enhances motivation and accountability, as individuals feel

connected to a larger fitness community regardless of their physical location.

3. **Innovative Training Modalities:**

The integration of technologies like virtual reality (VR) and augmented reality (AR) has opened up new possibilities in fitness. VR can immerse users in visually stunning environments, making workouts more enjoyable and engaging. AR overlays digital information onto the real world, providing users with real-time feedback and guidance during exercises. These innovations contribute to a more dynamic and personalized fitness experience.

4. **Wearable Technology and Fitness Trackers**:

Wearable devices, such as fitness trackers and smartwatches, play a crucial role in virtual fitness. These devices monitor various health metrics, track physical activity, and provide valuable data to users. The feedback from wearables allows individuals to set and track fitness goals, measure progress, and make informed decisions about their workouts and overall well-being.

5. **Personalization Algorithms**:

Virtual fitness platforms often employ sophisticated algorithms to personalize workout recommendations. These algorithms analyze user data, including fitness levels, preferences, and goals, to tailor workout plans. This personalized approach enhances the effectiveness of fitness routines, ensuring that individuals receive recommendations aligned with their specific needs and objectives.

6. **Global Connectivity for Fitness Professionals:**

Technology has enabled fitness professionals to connect with a global audience. Through virtual platforms, trainers and instructors can offer their expertise to clients worldwide. This global reach not only expands business opportunities for fitness professionals but also exposes users to diverse training styles, techniques, and cultural influences.

7. **Data-driven Insights**:

The integration of technology in virtual fitness generates a wealth of data. This data can provide valuable insights into user behavior, preferences, and performance. Fitness platforms can use this information to refine their offerings, improve user experiences, and develop more effective training programs.

While the impact of technology on virtual fitness is overwhelmingly positive, challenges such as the digital divide, potential privacy concerns, and the need for ongoing innovation to keep users engaged should be considered. Overall, technology continues to shape and enhance the virtual fitness landscape, making it an integral part of the modern approach to health and wellness.

ONLINE FITNESS CLASSES

Online fitness classes and platforms have experienced a surge in popularity, transforming the way individuals engage in physical activity and access professional guidance. The evolution of technology, coupled with the increasing demand for flexible and convenient workout options, has given rise to a diverse array of online fitness offerings. Here, we explore the key aspects and impacts of online fitness classes and platforms.

1. **Diversity of Offerings**:
   Online fitness platforms cater to a wide range of preferences and fitness levels. Users can choose from various types of workouts, including cardio, strength training, yoga, Pilates, dance, and more. This diversity allows individuals to explore different exercises and find routines that align with their interests and goals.

2. **Accessibility and Convenience:**

One of the primary advantages of online fitness classes is the unparalleled accessibility they offer. Users can participate in workouts from virtually anywhere, be it their homes, offices, or even while traveling. This convenience eliminates barriers such as commuting time and allows individuals to integrate fitness into their busy schedules.

3. **On-demand and Live Classes:**

Online fitness platforms typically provide two main formats: on-demand classes and live-streamed sessions. On-demand classes offer flexibility, enabling users to choose workouts at their preferred times. Live classes, on the other hand, create a sense of real-time engagement, as participants join instructors and fellow users from around the world in synchronized sessions.

4. **Interactivity and Community Building**:

Many online fitness platforms incorporate interactive features to enhance user engagement. Live chat, virtual high-fives, and social media integration create a sense of community, fostering motivation and accountability. This virtual camaraderie can be particularly beneficial for individuals who miss the social aspect of traditional gym classes.

5. **Expert Guidance and Personalization**:

Online fitness classes often feature experienced instructors and trainers who guide participants through workouts. Additionally, platforms leverage technology to personalize recommendations based on users' fitness levels, preferences, and goals. This combination of expert guidance and personalization enhances the effectiveness of virtual fitness experiences.

6. **Virtual Reality (VR) and Augmented Reality (AR):**

Some advanced online fitness platforms leverage VR and AR technologies to provide immersive and interactive experiences. VR can transport users to virtual environments, making workouts more engaging, while AR overlays digital information on the real world, offering guidance and feedback during exercises. These technologies contribute to a more dynamic and enjoyable fitness experience.

7. **Wearable Technology Integration:**

Wearable devices, such as fitness trackers and smartwatches, often integrate seamlessly with online fitness platforms. These devices can track users' performance, monitor vital signs, and provide real-time data during workouts. The integration of wearables enhances the overall fitness tracking and goal-setting capabilities of online platforms.

8. **Subscription Models and Free Content:**

Many online fitness platforms operate on subscription models, offering users access to a library of classes for a monthly fee. Some platforms, however, provide free content, allowing individuals to explore and try out workouts before committing to a subscription. This variety in pricing models caters to different user preferences and budget constraints.

In conclusion, online fitness classes and platforms have become integral to the modern fitness landscape. Their flexibility, accessibility, and diverse offerings make them a popular choice for individuals seeking convenient and personalized ways to stay active. As technology continues to advance, we can expect further innovations in online fitness, providing users with even more immersive and effective workout experiences.

PROS AND CONS OF VIRTUAL FITNESS EXPERIENCES

Virtual fitness experiences offer numerous benefits but also come with certain drawbacks. Here's an extensive exploration of the pros and cons:

Pros of Virtual Fitness Experiences:

1. **Accessibility**:
   - **Pro**: Virtual fitness provides easy access to workouts, eliminating geographical barriers. Individuals can exercise from the comfort of their homes, making fitness more accessible to a broader audience.

2. **Convenience**:
   - **Pro:** Users can choose when and where to work out, fitting sessions into their schedules without the need to commute to a physical location. This flexibility is particularly advantageous for those with busy lifestyles.

3. **Diverse Workout Options:**
   - **Pro:** Virtual platforms offer a wide variety of workout types, from traditional exercises to specialized programs like yoga, HIIT, dance, and more. Users can explore and find activities that match their preferences.

4. **Personalization**:
   - **Pro:** Many virtual fitness experiences use algorithms to personalize workouts based on individual preferences, fitness levels, and goals. This tailoring enhances the effectiveness of the exercise routine.

5. **Cost Savings**:

   - **Pro**: Virtual fitness can be cost-effective compared to traditional gym memberships. Users often pay a subscription fee for access to a diverse range of classes, eliminating the need for multiple memberships.

6. **Global Reach for Instructors**:

   - **Pro:** Fitness professionals can reach a global audience, expanding their client base beyond local limitations. This provides opportunities for trainers to connect with diverse groups of individuals.

7. **Innovative Technologies**:

   - **Pro:** Integration of technologies like virtual reality (VR) and augmented reality (AR) can enhance the overall workout experience, making it more engaging and enjoyable.

8. **Data Tracking and Analytics:**

   - **Pro**: Virtual fitness platforms often provide users with data and analytics related to their performance, helping individuals track progress and make informed decisions about their fitness journey.

Cons of Virtual Fitness Experiences:

1. **Lack of Physical Interaction**:
   - **Con**: Virtual fitness lacks the physical presence of instructors or workout partners, which can impact motivation and the sense of community. Some individuals thrive on the energy of in-person classes.

2. **Technical Issues**:
   - **Con:** Connectivity problems, software glitches, or device compatibility issues can disrupt virtual workouts. Technical challenges may hinder the overall experience and consistency of training.

3. **Motivational Challenges:**
   - **Con:** Some individuals may find it challenging to stay motivated without the social and competitive aspects of in-person fitness classes. The absence of real-time encouragement and feedback can be a drawback.

4. **Equipment Limitations:**
   - **Con**: Certain workouts may require specialized equipment that users may not have at home. While some virtual platforms offer equipment-free options, others may limit the variety of exercises available.

5. **Privacy Concerns**:

   - **Con:** Virtual workouts may raise privacy concerns, especially if users are uncomfortable with the idea of being monitored through cameras or sharing personal data on online platforms.

6. **Digital Fatigue:**

   - **Con:** The reliance on screens for work, socializing, and fitness can contribute to digital fatigue. Spending extended periods in virtual environments may negatively impact overall well-being.

7. **Limited Social Interaction:**

   - **Con:** The social aspect of traditional fitness classes is often lacking in virtual experiences. Building connections with instructors and fellow participants may be more challenging in an online setting.

8. **Quality Variability:**

   - **Con:** The quality of virtual fitness content can vary widely. While some platforms offer high-quality classes with experienced instructors, others may fall short, impacting the overall effectiveness of the workout.

In summary, virtual fitness experiences bring convenience, accessibility, and innovation to the world of exercise. However, they also pose challenges related to motivation, technology, and the absence of in-person interactions. The effectiveness of virtual fitness largely depends on individual preferences, goals, and adaptability to the digital exercise landscape.

CONCLUSION

In conclusion, the ever-evolving landscape of fitness is marked by several key trends that have significantly impacted how individuals approach and engage in physical activity. Let's recap some of the prominent trends discussed:

1. **Virtual Fitness Experiences:**
   - The rise of virtual fitness experiences has brought accessibility and convenience to the forefront. These platforms leverage technology to offer a diverse range of workouts, personalized training, and even immersive experiences through technologies like virtual and augmented reality.

2. **Online Fitness Classes and Platforms**:
   - Online fitness classes have become immensely popular, providing users with flexibility and the

ability to choose from a variety of workouts. The integration of technology, wearable devices, and interactive features has enhanced the overall fitness experience.

Reflecting on these trends, it's clear that the fitness industry is leveraging technology to cater to the diverse needs and preferences of individuals. Whether through virtual workouts, online classes, or innovative technologies, the goal is to make fitness more accessible, engaging, and personalized.

As we navigate this dynamic landscape, it's essential to recognize that there is no one-size-fits-all approach to fitness. Encouraging readers to explore different trends, classes, and technologies is crucial. What works for one person may not work for another, and discovering the right fit is a personal journey.

Embracing technology-enhanced fitness experiences doesn't mean abandoning traditional forms of exercise or the pursuit of physical activities outside of the digital realm. The key is to find a balance that aligns with individual preferences, goals, and lifestyles.

In the quest for a healthier and more active lifestyle, individuals are encouraged to:

- **Explore Varied Workouts**: Try different types of workouts to discover what resonates most, whether it's high-intensity interval training (HIIT), yoga, strength training, or dance workouts.

- **Stay Open to Innovation:** Embrace technological advancements in fitness, such as virtual reality, augmented reality, and wearable devices. These innovations can add a new dimension to workouts and make the fitness journey more enjoyable.

- **Listen to Your Body**: Pay attention to how your body responds to different forms of exercise. Finding activities that you enjoy and that align with your fitness goals can make the journey more sustainable and fulfilling.

- **Connect with Community:** Whether online or in-person, building connections with like-minded individuals can provide motivation and support. Engaging in group activities or classes fosters a sense of community, enhancing the overall fitness experience.

In conclusion, the world of fitness is dynamic, offering a multitude of options to cater to diverse preferences and lifestyles. By staying open to exploration, embracing innovation, and finding joy in the process, individuals can embark on a fitness journey that is not only effective but also enjoyable and sustainable. The key is to make fitness a personalized and rewarding part of one's lifestyle.

www.ingramcontent.com/pod-product-compliance
Lightning Source LLC
Chambersburg PA
CBHW071609270726
48661CB00019B/1675